The Ultimate Cures And Remedies For Hair Loss

The Most Effective, Permanent Solution to Finally Stop Hair Loss And Prevent Balding For Life

John K.

Table of Contents

Check Out My Other Books

Introduction

I want to thank you and congratulate you for purchasing the book, *"The Ultimate Cures And Remedies For Hair Loss: The Most Effective, Permanent Solution to Finally Stop Hair Loss And Prevent Balding For Life"*.

A full head of hair is associated with strength, virility, youth, and power. Unexplained, excessive hair loss can be worrying and scary. The good news is, there are different ways to fix it. This book contains proven steps and strategies on how to control your hair loss and understanding the facts associated with it. Also covers different diseases related to hair and scalp and methods to overcome it. We will learn about hair, Diet and nutrition needed for proper hair, Grooming techniques, Hair and Scalp diseases, and Some advanced techniques for restoring hair and finally the medications.

Thanks again for purchasing this book. I hope you enjoy it!

The information herein is offered for informational purposes solely, and is universal as so. The presentation of the information is without contract or any type of guarantee assurance.

The trademarks that are used are without any consent, and the publication of the trademark is without permission or backing by the trademark owner. All trademarks and brands within this book are for clarifying purposes only and are the owned by the owners themselves, not affiliated with this document.

Chapter 1 - Hair Facts and Hair Loss Basics

Hair is the fastest growing tissue of the body, made up of proteins called keratins. Every strand of hair is made up of three layers: the inner layer or medulla (only present in thick hairs); the middle layer or cortex, which determines the strength, texture, and color of hair; and the cuticle, which protects the cortex. Hair grows from roots, which are enclosed in follicles. Below this is a layer of skin called the dermal papilla, which is fed by the bloodstream carrying nourishments vital to the growth of hair. Only the roots of hair are actually alive, while the visible part of hair is dead tissue, and therefore unable to heal itself. It is vital then to take care of the scalp and body in order to perpetuate hair growth and maintenance. Expensive treatments that claim to treat the visible hair and nourish it therefore are usually no more than bogus claims made to sell products.

Hormones called androgens, usually testosterone, can cause hair follicles to shrink, causing thinning of hair or eventual hair loss. Reportedly only bone marrow grows faster in our body than hair does. The average scalp contains 100,000-150,000 hair follicles and hairs, with 90% growing and 10% resting at any given time. Hair actually grows in three stages: anagen, catagen, and telogen. The anagen phase is the phase where hair is actively growing, and of course this phase is longer for follicles in the scalp than anywhere else on your body, and lasts longer for women than men. It is natural for follicles to atrophy and hair to fall out, and this is called the catagen phase. This phase is only temporary, and eventually the follicle enters the telogen phase where it is resting. These are the 10% at rest mentioned above. Normal anagen phases last approximately five years, with catagen phases lasting about three weeks, and telogen phases lasting approximately 12 weeks. As you see it is natural to lose some hair. Natural hair loss is considered to be in the range of 100 hairs per day. It is not apparent to most people that hair is actually being lost until more than 50% of a person's hair is actually lost.

Although both men and women can suffer significant hair loss, over 50% of men will suffer with Male Pattern Baldness (MPB), also known as androgenetic alopecia, at some point in their lives. The reason behind hair loss is a genetically inherited sensitivity to Dihydrotestosterone (DHT) and 5-alpha-reductase. The enzyme 5-alpha-reductase converts testosterone, a male hormone, to DHT, the substance identified as the end-cause for hair loss.

Most hair loss follows a pattern that has been codified in a table called the Norwood Scale (see figure 1). There are seven patterns of hair identified in the Norwood Scale,

a) Norwood I being a normal head of hair with no visible hair loss,

b) Norwood II showing the hair receding in a wedge-shaped pattern.

c) Norwood III shows the same receding pattern as Norwood II, except the hairline has receded deeper into the frontal area and the temporal area.

d) Type IV on the Norwood Scale indicates a hairline that has receded more dramatically in the frontal region and temporal area. Additionally there is a balding area at the very top center of the head, but there is a bridge of hair remaining between that region and the front.

e) Type V on the Norwood Scale shows that very same bridge between the frontal region and the top center, also called the vertex, beginning to thin.

f) Type VI on the Norwood Scale indicates that the bridge between the frontal region and the vertex has disappeared.

g) Finally, Type VII on the Norwood Scale shows hair receding all the way back to the base of the head and the sides just above the ears.

Norwood patterns are determined genetically.

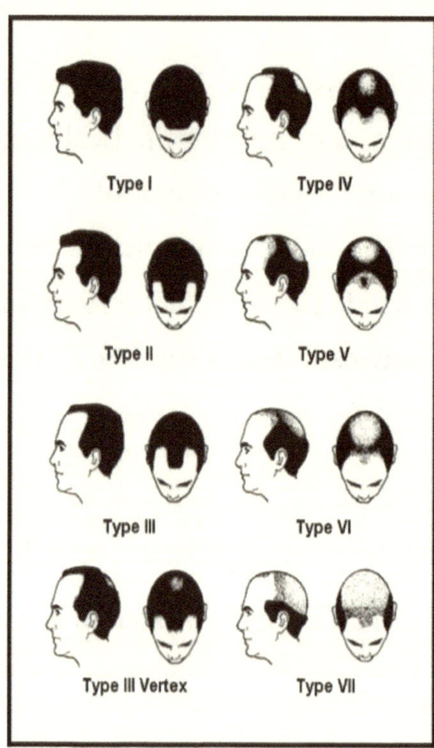

Figure 1. Norwood Scale

Interesting Study

Hair loss has been noticed and studied throughout the ages, and some interesting discoveries were made in ancient times. For one it was noticed that eunuchs: those males without genitals-never went bald. Men who were castrated as a result of accidents in battle also never went bald. This was the first indication that testosterone had something to do with hair loss. It has also been found that the more recessive the hair gene, the more propensity toward baldness one has. Blond-haired persons have a greater propensity toward hair loss than darker-haired people, and therefore Caucasian persons have a greater propensity toward hair loss than non-Caucasian people. Beyond the genetic propensity of certain people toward hair loss, there seems to be various dietary triggers that activate the process, a notion that is promising since this can be controlled.

Androgens

What exactly are androgens? Androgens are sex hormones mainly produced by males, the main one of which is testosterone. Androgens are produced by the adrenal glands, which protect the body in stressful situations by also producing adrenaline so that the body may respond to situations it deems to be threatening. The stress of daily life in Western civilization has caused a state of alarm in people that has made the body unable to distinguish between everyday stressors and threatening situations. Therefore the adrenal glands in most people in Western civilizations are overactive, constantly producing adrenaline and naturally producing testosterone along with it. Additionally, the over-consumption of red meat and high fat foods in Western society cause an overactive adrenal gland, perpetuating this situation.

There is a definite connection between the syndrome of Male Pattern Baldness (MPB) and the prostate gland. The prostate gland is actually a cluster of small glands in males surrounding the urethra, located just below the bladder. There is not a lot known about all the functions of the prostate, except that it serves to squeeze seminal fluid into and through the urethra during ejaculation. Prostate problems can cause serious problems with urination it becomes enlarged, and sometimes the prostate becomes cancerous. The syndrome of non-cancerous enlargement of the prostate is known as benign prostatic hyperplasia (BPH). DHT is responsible for the division of cells in the prostate, and is normally expelled by the prostate. However, when the prostate fails to expel the DHT, it builds up and causes enlargement. It has been confirmed that typical North American and northern European diets lend to the perpetuation of BPH and prostate cancer, whereas these are uncommon phenomena in other lands and was even uncommon here in the past. This is significant because the overproduction of DHT is responsible for BPH and prostate cancer, and is also responsible for MPB or androgenetic alopecia. The findings in research for BPH cures have usually simultaneously produced benefits in hair growth. We shall cover some of these discoveries in various sections of this book. Additionally, changes in diet are necessary to avoid all of these conditions and improve overall health.

Some common myths have arisen concerning hair loss. Because of medical advancements many of these myths are being addressed and corrected. For starters, although androgenetic alopecia or pattern baldness is genetic and therefore can be hereditary, it is not passed down through only your mother's side of the family. Either side of the family can pass down the genetic disposition toward baldness. Also, contrary to old family tales, wearing hats does not cause baldness either. Most common hair loss comes under what has been commonly known as Male Pattern Baldness (MPB). Although referred to as MPB, females suffer a similar syndrome, so it is more properly called androgenetic alopecia. Although hair loss is not life or health threatening, it can cause serious problems with a person's psyche and self- confidence. There has been no absolute cure found for hair loss, and many factors of hair loss are hereditary, however there are several preventative measures one can take to maintain healthy hair and scalp.

Chapter 2 - Diet, Nutrition and Hair Loss

Healthy Diet for Healthy Hair

One key factor in maintaining a growing protein on a part of one's biological body is obvious: one must maintain a healthy diet. Although certain factors have been definitely identified as contributors to hair loss, we must keep in mind that hair is part of the complete biological system of the human body. Being a system, dysfunctions in one part of the system can contribute to dysfunctions in other parts; chain reactions occur when one part of the body malfunctions, causing other parts within the system to falter. To maintain optimum health, it is best to maintain a healthy diet and regular exercise regimen.

Defining exactly what a healthy diet is when it comes to preventing hair loss can be a little more complex. Principally, the main vitamins, minerals, and nutrients that one must ingest in some form to maintain healthy hair are vitamin A, all B vitamins- particularly vitamins B-6 and B-12, folic acid, biotin, vitamin C, vitamin E, copper, iron, zinc, iodine, protein of course, silica, essential fatty acids (EFA's, formerly known as vitamin F) and last but not least one must consume water. There are also certain foods that may cause dysfunctions that will contribute to hair loss. The best way to maintain a healthy vitamin and mineral intake is a good diet. It is not necessary or advisable to go out and buy a bunch of over-the-counter vitamin supplements in order to achieve your suggested nutritional levels. Many over-the-counter vitamins are chemically processed and are not completely absorbed into the system. It is also easy to overdose oneself with over the counter vitamins particularly when taking supplements of fat-soluble vitamins and minerals, causing toxicity and adverse reactions. The likelihood of doing this is far less with food; therefore it is always best to obtain the bulk of your vitamin and mineral re□uirements from whole foods.

1. Vitamin A

Vitamin A is a key component to developing healthy cells and tissues in the body, including hair. Additionally it works with silica and zinc to prevent drying and clogging of the sebaceous glands, the glands vital to producing sebum, which is an important lubricant for the hair follicle. Vitamin A deficiencies commonly cause thickening of the scalp, dry hair, and dandruff. Air pollution, smoking, extremely bright light, certain cholesterol-lowering drugs, laxatives, and aspirin are some known vitamin A inhibitors. Liver, fish oil, eggs, fortified milk, and red, yellow, and orange vegetables are good sources for vitamin A, as are some dark green leafy vegetables like spinach. Be particularly careful if you take vitamin A supplements, as vitamin A is fat-soluble, allowing the body to store it and making it easy for the body to overdose on vitamin A. Vitamin A overdoses can cause excessively dry skin and inflamed hair follicles, and in some cases ironically can cause hair loss. If you choose to take supplements of this vitamin, consult with a specialist first. As mentioned above, the likelihood of overdosing by achieving your vitamin A intake by food sources is almost nil, so it is best to attempt to achieve this at all costs.

2. Vitamin B

B-vitamins work interdependently and therefore all levels of B vitamins need to be sufficient in order to maintain proper health. Vitamins B-6, folic acid, biotin, and vitamin B-12 are all key components in maintaining healthy hemoglobin levels in the blood, which is the iron-containing portion of red-blood cells. Hemoglobin's primary function is to carry oxygen from the lungs to the tissues of the body, so if these vitamins were deficient in one's body, then hair and skin would indeed suffer. Fortunately some of the tastiest foods contain these vitamins. Vitamin B-6 is found in protein rich foods, which is excellent because the body needs a sufficient amount of protein to maintain hair growth as well. Liver, chicken, fish, pork, kidney, and soybeans are good sources of B-6 and are relatively low in fat when they are not fried. Folic acid is found in whole grains, cereals, nuts, green leafy vegetables, orange juice, brewer's yeast, wheat germ, and liver again. Meat, fish, poultry, eggs, and other dairy products meanwhile provide healthy amounts of B-12. Biotin deficiencies are rare unless there is a severe case of malnutrition or a serious intestinal disorder, since a healthy gut produces biotin through good bacteria found there. Note: if you have a known intestinal disorder and are plagued by hair loss, ask your doctor about biotin deficiencies and possible solutions.

3. Vitamin C

Vitamin C is responsible for the development of healthy collagen, which is necessary to hold body tissues together. A vitamin C deficiency can cause split ends and hair breakage, yet this is easily reversible with an increase to normal vitamin C levels. Vitamin C can be found in foods such as fresh peppers, citrus fruits, melons berries, potatoes, tomatoes, and dark green leafy vegetables.

4. Vitamin E

Vitamin E is necessary to provide good blood circulation to the scalp by increasing the uptake of oxygen. Vitamin E is derived from foods such as green leafy vegetables, nuts, grains, vegetable oils, and most ready-to-eat cereals, which are fortified with vitamin E. Vitamin E deficiencies are rare in people in North America and Europe. In the rare cases of vitamin E deficiency, usually caused by the inability to absorb oils and fats, dietary supplements are available.

5. Copper

Copper is a trace mineral that is also necessary in the production of hemoglobin. Hemoglobin as mentioned earlier is vital to the process of carrying oxygen to tissues such as the hair, and obviously hair is alive cannot grow without proper oxygen, yet it does not breathe as other components of our body do, because the oxygen must get to the shaft of the hair. Good sources of copper are liver again, seafood, nuts, and seeds.

6. Iron

Another key mineral vital in the production of hemoglobin is iron. Iron is found in two forms, heme and non-heme; heme iron is much easier to absorb into the system. This is where the problem lies. Of course most people know that red meat is a good source of iron, however red meat is non-heme iron and is difficult for the body to absorb, as are many iron supplements. Good heme iron sources are green leafy vegetables, kidney beans, and bran. Additionally, one can increase the absorption of non-heme iron into the body by consuming non-heme food sources and vitamin C sources in the same meal.

7. Zinc

Zinc is another vital component to healthy hair, being that it is responsible for cell production, tissue growth and repair, and the maintenance of the oil-secreting glands of the scalp. It also plays a large role in protein synthesis and collagen formation. For this reason, zinc is important for both hair maintenance and dandruff prevention. Most Americans are deficient in zinc. Most foods of animal origin, particularly seafood, contain good amounts of zinc; oysters are particularly rich in zinc. Zinc is also found in eggs and milk, although in much smaller amounts. Zinc from sources such as nuts, legumes, and natural grains is of a different type than those found in animal sources and is not easily used by the body, although oats are a good source of zinc that is readily used by the body.

8. Protein

Protein is found in most of the aforementioned animal source foods, particularly meats, fish, milk, cheese, eggs and yogurt. There is no need for a person eating the average Western diet to eat additional protein. Too much protein, even though hair is made of protein, will not improve hair growth and may cause other health problems. A challenge for vegans is to maintain healthy levels of protein, being that complete proteins containing all nine essential amino acids necessary are found mostly in animal sources. Legumes, seeds, nuts, grains and vegetables do not contain the same form of protein necessary for a healthy body. There is only one common non-meat source for complete protein, and that is the soybean. Fortunately, soybeans have been made into tofu and texturized vegetable protein (TVP) so that they can be made into various dishes. Additionally, one may eat from a wide variety of vegetable sources in order to obtain all the essential amino acids.

9. Iodine

Iodine is vital to the growth of hair. Sheep farmers long ago discovered that vegetation void of iodine due to iodine-depleted soil will adversely affect the growth of wool in sheep. Likewise, our hair needs iodine to grow. Iodine is synthetically added to table salt, however in this form it is not assimilated well into the body and can therefore cause iodine overload. An excess of iodine in the body can adversely affect the thyroid. It is best to use non-iodized salt and retrieve your iodine from natural food sources. These include seaweed, salmon, seafood, lima beans, molasses, eggs, potatoes with the skin on, watercress and garlic. One of the most difficult nutrients vital to hair growth to get in one's diet is the trace mineral silica.

10.   Silicon

Silicon is a form of silicon and is the second most abundant element in the earth's crust, second only to oxygen. The Earth provides everything we need for health, and with silicon being so abundant, it would seem that there would never be a problem with silica deficiency. Unfortunately, trace minerals are rare in Western diets because our food is processed and our soil depleted by chemical treatments so often that trace minerals are lost. Silica is vital to the strength of hair, and although it will not necessarily stop hair from falling out from the follicle, it will stop hair breakage. It works by stimulating the cell metabolism and formation, which slows the aging process. Foods that are rich in silica are rice, oats, lettuce, parsnips, asparagus, onion, strawberry, cabbage, cucumber, leek, sunflower seeds, celery, rhubarb, cauliflower, and swiss chard. Note that many of these foods, particularly rice, are a large part of Asian diets and Asians tend to have the strongest and healthiest hair. Be sure to seek out all the above foods from sources that grow food organically, as this is vital to obtaining the trace minerals that are usually not present in North American soil and therefore not in American foods. Additionally these foods should be eaten uncooked, or in the case of rice-unwashed, as trace minerals are easily cooked and washed away.

11. Essential Fatty Acids(EFA's)

Essential Fatty Acids (EFA's) are fatty acids that are needed by the body yet not produced by the body. EFA's are a key component to healthy skin, hair and nails. Common skin diseases, such as those discussed later in this book like eczema and seborrhea, are in part caused by deficiencies in EFA's. Including deep-water fish such as salmon, sardines, mackerel, trout, or herring approximately three times a week will provide sufficient amounts of EFA's. However, if for some reason you cannot eat deep- water fish or have an extreme dislike for it, it may be necessary to take a supplement to obtain the required amount of EFA's.

12. Water

Last but not least, make sure to include the proper amount of water in your diet. Water is vital to proper hydration, which is necessary in order for all nutrients to be utilized properly by the body, not to mention the proper function of every cell in the body including hair follicles. The suggested amount of water intake daily is eight 8-ounce glasses of water a day, or 64 ounces a day.

13. Lower the consumption of High-Fat diets

The effects of high-fat diets and the increase of DHT (Dihydrotestosterone), a chemical produced by the body found to cause hair loss, is not conclusive at this time. However, there does seem to be a connection; as societies that consumed relatively low- fat diets such as pre-World War II Japan experienced almost no pattern baldness, whereas in post-World War II Japan there is an increase in pattern baldness as their society consumes a higher fat diet. In fact, Asian and African men in their native countries traditionally suffer very little Male Pattern Baldness (MPB). Although when the same peoples come to North America, they begin to develop MPB. Because people of all races and ethnicities tend to develop MPB or androgenetic alopecia, yet do not exhibit these tendencies before moving to America, changes in diet may be a leading contributing factor. Diets high in fat do increase testosterone, which is the main component in DHT. More research needs to be done on this topic to reach conclusive evidence, although it certainly could not hurt to lower one's fat intake.

14. Fiber

Fiber is vital to making sure undigested food moves through the body and to the bowels properly. Failure of foods to move through the bowels in a reasonable amount of time can cause fermentation of undigested food in the bowels and blocking of nutrients being absorbed through the body. Beyond causing degrees of malnutrition, this can also cause a level of toxicity that will overwork systems in the body such as the adrenal glands and contribute to hair loss. Healthy amounts of fresh vegetables, fruits and legumes consumed daily will ensure a proper amount of dietary fiber.

Supplements

Although nutritional remedies were those that were discussed here, supplements can be used if one feels they are simply unable to eat properly due to work schedule or dislike of certain foods. Nutritional supplements containing these same vitamins and minerals can be taken, with the exception of water of course. Be sure to always take supplements that are naturally chelated, meaning that the supplements were developed in a natural base. This will ensure that the supplements you consume will be more readily absorbed in the body. There are some cautions to taking supplements of certain vitamins and minerals, particularly those that are fat-soluble because the body stores them.

Vitamin A can be highly toxic and supplements of vitamin A should be avoided unless recommended by a doctor. It is best to achieve one's vitamin A requirements either by food or through a naturally chelated multivitamin. Also remember that smoking and second hand smoke can cause blocking of vitamin A assimilation, so it is best to avoid smoking and remove one's self from areas and situations where second hand smoke is present if at all possible.

Vitamin E supplements should always be taken at 400 i.u. per day to start and work your way up to 800 i.u. Always take vitamin E in its natural form, which is d'alpha tocopherol. Avoid taking vitamin E supplements in the synthetic form dl'alpha tocopherol, which is derived from petroleum and is less available for assimilation into the body. If you have high blood pressure or other serious illnesses, consult a physician before taking vitamin E supplements.

Zinc is one fat-soluble mineral that can cause harm if an overdose is taken. Zinc can rob the body of copper, mentioned above as a key nutrient in hair growth and health, not to mention in other functions of the body. Zinc supplements should be taken in low doses, such as 5mg at a time. These can commonly be found in the form of zinc lozenges designed for sore throats. There is a "trick" to tell if you are taking too much zinc. When the zinc levels in the body have surpassed the level that they can be used, a metallic taste begins to form. If you pay attention to the metallic taste, you will know when enough zinc has been consumed, and you can then stop consuming zinc immediately.

Iron supplements are not recommended unless a doctor has diagnosed you with a severe iron deficiency. If you do take an iron supplement, avoid ferrous sulfate, which you will find as the most common over-the-counter iron supplement in drug stores.

Ferrous sulfate is hard for the body to assimilate, and because iron is not water-soluble it will sit in the body and can cause severe liver problems over time. Further, ferrous sulfate causes constipation, which can trigger a great deal more problems besides being extremely unpleasant. One iron supplement that does not contain ferrous sulfate is called Floradix and is available in both liquid and pill form.

Since there are so few foods to mention that are grown in North America and contain a good amount of silica, supplements may truly be needed. Horsetail is an herb that is a rich source of silica. It is highly important to never take horsetail directly however, or take a supplement made from unprocessed horsetail, as this herb can be toxic when ingested whole, ground, in tablets or capsules. Horsetail must be taken in an aqueous extract of the herb only. Ask someone at your health food store or someone knowledgeable about herbs to help you find this form. Silica gel is suspended in water, although it is not an aqueous solution and should be avoided. Nettle is also a good source of silica and Nettle Root Extract is readily available at health food stores.

Supplements of Essential Fatty Acids (EFA's) are easily found in most health food stores and even many supermarkets and pharmacies. These include Evening Primrose Oil, Wheat Germ Oil, Flaxseed Oil, Cod Liver Oil, and other oils from deep- water fish. It is not recommended to rely on Cod Liver Oil as a source for EFA's because it contains high levels of vitamins A and D, and the amount of Cod Liver Oil necessary to achieve proper amounts of EFA's would cause overdosing on these vitamins. The recommended supplements are Evening Primrose Oil and Flaxseed Oil. Both these oils are available in oil form or in capsules. Keep in mind that high amounts of saturated fat blocks the effectiveness of EFA's, counteracting their effectiveness, so there needs to be adjustments to your diet if there is a high amount of saturated fat in it.

Juicing

Juicing is a natural way to obtain many of the vitamins, minerals, and trace minerals mentioned above. When using organic fruits and vegetables, juicing can provide quite a boost to the system and encourage the health of hair. Juices are very readily assimilable by the body and provide the same content as the whole food. Fresh juices have a high enzyme content, which is beneficial because these enzymes are stored by the body and can be used by the body when cooked foods that have been robbed of enzymes are consumed.

Storing the juice or purchasing pasteurized juices from the store diminishes this benefit, although the benefits of the minerals and vitamins are usually still available. All the above-mentioned fruits and vegetables can be juiced to obtain the maximum benefit from them.

A great deal of silica, sulfur, iron, and potassium for example is extracted from organic carrot juice. In fact, carrots being roots contain most trace minerals the body needs. The effects of carrot juice are enhanced when adding cucumber juice to it, because of its high silica and sulfur content.

Organic spinach juice is highly recommended, as it is high in iron, vitamin A, and other vital vitamins and minerals; it is often combined with lettuce and carrot juice, two very good sources of silica and vitamin A.

Non-organic spinach juice can be extremely high in pesticides and should therefore be avoided. Spinach juice should also be avoided if one suffers from kidney stones, as it contains a large amount of oxalic acid, which exacerbates kidney stone growth.

Foods to avoid

There are a number of foods and substances to avoid and limit the intake of.

Substances such as alcohol, caffeine, sugar and nicotine can deplete the body of nutrients and raise adrenal levels, which will cause a chain reaction of producing more androgen and causing hair loss.

High levels of saturated fat and cholesterol rich foods are also linked to increased DHT levels and their consumption should be limited.

Additionally, common table salt has been linked to hair loss. And the average diet provides the recommended amount of sodium intake; therefore, salt should never be added to food. However, when using salt for seasoning during cooking, be sure to use salt with Iodine being that it is a nutrient that is vital to hair growth as well, unless you are a regular consumer of seafood, which contains high levels of Iodine.

Toxemia can cause a great deal of dysfunction in the body's systems, including hair-loss related illnesses such as eczema, psoriasis, seborrhea and possibly several others. It is vital for one to cleanse the body of impurities in order to maintain a healthy system and avoid such illnesses, as there are no cure for these illnesses beyond cleansing and the maintenance of a healthy diet to allow the body to heal itself.

Regular cleansing should include a diet rich in fiber as mentioned earlier, and the use of added fiber such as provided by consuming psyllium husk as a bulking agent along with laxative agents. More is discussed under the section Natural Hair Loss Remedies.

Although hair loss can be caused by many other variables, lack of proper nutrition will assuredly cause hair loss in many people. Fortunately, adopting a proper diet that includes the above nutrients can reverse hair loss caused by malnutrition. One thing for certain, regardless of whether your hair loss was caused by malnutrition or not, adopting a healthier diet will help the function of other areas of the body.

Chapter 3 - Natural Hair Loss Remedies

There is again no sure-fire way to prevent all hair loss; however, there are some methods that have been used that work on some people.

Naturopathic Remedy

In addition to the dietary improvements and suggestions already offered, there are some naturopathic remedy suggestions.

1. Massage and Aromatherapy

Massage and aromatherapy have been used with some success. In minor cases of temporary hair loss, hair growth can be stimulated by massage, since blood and oxygen flow to the scalp must be healthy in order for hair to grow.

A blend of six drops each of lavender and bay essential oils in a base of four ounces of either almond, soybean or sesame oil massaged into the scalp and allowed to sit for 20 minutes has been used by aroma therapists to stimulate the scalp. Once the mixture is in the scalp for 20 minutes, wash your hair and scalp with your normal shampoo mixed with three drops of bay essential oil.

Massaging the scalp in general for a couple of minutes a day can stimulate blood flow to the hair follicles and in mild cases stimulate some hair growth. Of course, one must be careful to be gentle when massaging and not tug at the hair or use the fingernails when massaging the scalp. If one is concerned about fingernails getting in the way due to extra long fingernails, there are several options. One is a flat-handed massage, which while not as effective as the finger massage can provide some circulatory benefits and results.

There are several electric massagers on the market that have an attachment for scalp massaging as well. An oriental method called Qi Gong (pronounced Chi Kung) has been used to increase circulation to the scalp and face also. The fingers should be placed at the center of the skull base and then begin to tap approximately 30 times. Work your way outward toward the ears continuing to tap gently. After reaching the ears go back to the center of the skull a little higher up and work your way around to the ear region. Keep going up about eight levels, each time repeating the process.

2. herb Saw Palmetto

As mentioned earlier, there is a definite connection between the prostate and hair loss for men, and therefore a connection between breakthroughs in BPH treatments developed and their effectiveness in restoring hair growth. There have been some herbalists that have experimented with the herb Saw Palmetto in order to block the production of DHT in treating BPH. Although most studies of Saw Palmetto have been for the treatment of prostatic disease, more recent studies have been conducted on its effectiveness in treating loss. The herb has been found to work in fighting benign prostatic disease by lowering levels of DHT, which is a known cause of androgenetic alopecia. Studies have shown Saw Palmetto extract is an effective anti-androgen and therefore there is promise for its effectiveness as an effective treatment for hair loss prevention. Women who take Saw Palmetto should cease doing so when taking oral contraceptives or hormone therapy.

3. Nettles Root Extract

Nettles are rich in vitamins A and C, several key minerals and lipids that can be beneficial to the hair. Nettle Root Extract has been used successfully in Europe as an inhibitor of 5-alpha reductase in treating BPH. As mentioned earlier, 5-alpha reductase is a key component in turning testosterone into DHT, the substance that causes the atrophy of hair follicles. Therefore there is great promise in its use as a component in natural hair loss treatments. Nettle Root Extract is available at health food stores over the counter, and has few side effects.

4. Rosemary and Sage

Rosemary and sage are two herbs that have shown benefit traditionally when used externally. It is suggested that to promote a clean scalp, stimulation of the hair root, and thickening hair one should boil together in water rosemary, sage, peach leaf, nettle and burdock. Then strain the loose herbs from the liquid and use the liquid to wash the hair daily. Also recommended is steeping one ounce of ground rosemary, two ounces of ground sage, and a half ounce of ground nettles in one pint of ethyl alcohol for a week, straining the solution and adding one ounce of castor oil and one ounce of water to the liquid. This is said to make a great hair lotion to apply at night before bed or just before shampooing.

5. Jojoba

If one is predisposed to seborrhea, eczema, psoriasis, or dandruff, one might consider the use of jojoba (pronounced ho-ho-ba) oil. Mexicans and southwestern Native American nations have used jojoba oil traditionally for centuries to promote hair growth and the control of dandruff. Jojoba oil is great for hypoallergenic skin by being a great moisturizer and mimicking the scalp's own sebum. It absorbs readily into the scalp and helps remove deposits of sebum from the hair follicles, neutralizes acidity, and nourishes the scalp with all the B vitamins, vitamin E, silicon, copper, zinc, chromium, and iodine.

6. Aloe Vera

Aloe Vera has been used by Native Americans, Indians and many in the Caribbean to promote healthy hair and prevent hair loss. Aloe's positive effects on the skin are well known, and likewise it can help the scalp by healing it and balancing the pH level of the scalp while cleansing the pores. A common preparation of Aloe Vera gel with a small amount of wheat germ oil and coconut milk is used as a shampoo and has traditionally shown great benefit. Of course, if you do not want to go through the trouble of concocting your own formulas, similar products or products containing these ingredients may be found in the health food store if one does some searching.

7. Using Henna

While Henna will not promote hair growth, henna is excellent for the maintenance of healthy hair. Henna is a natural clay conditioner that can help heal the hair shaft by repairing and sealing the cuticle, protecting hair against breakage and loss of shine. Henna comes in a variety of colors to safely color or highlight the hair temporarily, or one can obtain neutral henna if one does not desire color changes to the hair.

8. Cleansing

Cleansing should be a major part of your regimen to maintain and grow hair. Many scalp related diseases are directly the result of toxemia, while toxins in the body adversely affecting the body's systems indirectly affect other conditions. Cleansing should be performed through oral means regularly and occasionally by enema or colonic irrigation; and the colon is the key to health and the root of nearly all of the body's illnesses. A clogged colon blocks the ability of the body to absorb nutrients from foods you consume, therefore causing possible malnutrition of the hair. When the colon is clogged, toxins are harbored that harm the body. Excess toxins send the body into a panic and overwork other organs of the body when the colon cannot eliminate them. Commonly overworked organs are the liver and the kidneys, however the trickle-down effect actually causes the adrenal glands to overproduce testosterone, leading to increased levels of DHT.

9. Polysorbate-80

Polysorbate-80 is an FDA approved surfactant that is also approved as a food additive. It causes water and oils or fats to mix, and according to research, is of very little toxicity. Although it is not proven, Polysorbate-80 is said to remove deposits of DHT and cholesterol from the scalp. Polysorbate-80 is a common additive in shampoo and is also available in its stand-alone form inn health food stores. It is being recommended by some naturopathic practitioners as an application for the scalp approximately 15 minutes prior to shampooing.

10.   Fiber rich food(Psyllium Husk)

Fiber is vital to cleansing, and most North American diets are deficient in natural fiber. Psyllium husk is a bulking laxative agent that can be used to safely move waste through the colon. Psyllium is a very good substance as it gently scrubs the walls of the colon to remove waste that is stuck to the walls. Activating agents such as the herbs cascara sagrada, senna and cayenne help activate the peristaltic waves of the intestines to push clogged waste through the colon and out. It would be best to consult an herbalist, naturopath or purchase a prepared herbal tea containing the aforementioned herbs. However, the psyllium can be obtained from any health food store and mixed with water. Be sure to drink the psyllium as soon as you mix it as it will begin to turn into a gel-like substance that will be harder to swallow. Psyllium has no taste, and although many do not like its gritty feeling, the benefits far outweigh the unpleasantness.

11. Colonic Irrigation

Occasionally, a full colonic irrigation should be sought from a licensed professional. Colonic irrigations clean the colon through the gentle application of water into the colon by a colonic irrigation machine. Licensed practitioners who perform this function are available in most states and the benefits are unequalled. Commonly called a colonic for short, this process can remove far more waste than cleansing by taking herbs orally. With a proper diet, one should only need to have a colonic seasonally or even as little as bi-annually, for those who are maintaining a high-fiber diet. For the first treatment however, one should go through a series of colonic irrigation cleansings, since waste is impacted in the colon and must be gradually loosened. Once one has cleansed internally, cleanliness must be maintained to avoid the buildup of toxins reoccurring.

12. Detoxifying Herbal Teas

Detoxifying herbal teas such as saffron are gentle and can be drunk to remove toxins from the body. Saffron has the effect of carrying toxins from inside the body out through the pores of the skin. Chamomile, mullein or watermelon seed tea can be substituted for saffron tea for this purpose. This process is assisted by utilizing a steam bath to open the pores to allow toxins to come out easier. Be sure to consume plenty of fluids such as water and sports drinks that contain salts your body may lose before entering a steam bath. Steam baths are extremely beneficial, yet your body will lose a large amount of water and salt, so you want to be sure to consume extra amounts of water and salt before going into the steam bath, and keep some sports drinks on hand in case you feel depleted. Of course if you have any medical conditions that affect your stamina, endurance, blood pressure, or breathing, consult your physician before engaging in steam baths.

13. Exercises

Finally, although exercise does absolutely nothing directly to grow hair, most holistic practitioners when questioned about hair loss recommend it. The reason was stated earlier, that being the fact that the body is a complete system, and neglect of the system can cause chain reactions of which one result may be hair loss. Take some time to exercise daily if only for a few minutes. This will improve blood flow, the delivery of oxygen to the cells of the body, and help the digestion of foods, all things that aid the health of hair follicles. If you have access to seawater, swimming is one of the most complete exercises available. It exercises the entire body with little stress on the joints, and the seawater helps wash away toxins. However, beware of swimming in chlorinated water such as found in most pools, as chlorine can have negative effects on the hair. Bicycling is also another low-impact beneficial exercise that can be done in one's neighborhood or on a stationary bicycle, as is walking. Whatever method of exercising you choose, simply exercise to improve overall health. In combination with the other methods presented here, exercise will only help your condition.

Chapter 4 - Good Grooming and Care

Hair is fairly strong and can generally withstand normal grooming techniques. However, there can be thinning or breakage of hair due to poor grooming habits, and following several tips can prevent these bouts of thinning and breakage.

1. Avoid combing hair When wet

Avoid combing hair with fine-toothed combs when wet, as this is a common cause of breakage. Although this is a tempting practice because hair straightens and detangles much better if combed when wet, the stress on the hair shaft is immense when the hair is wet because it is weakened.

2. Avoid Brushing of hair when wet

This goes for brushing the hair when wet also. Brushing the hair in general can be stimulating to the scalp, encouraging blood flow to the hair follicles and maintaining their health. Brushing the hair before washing it can loosen up flakes of sebum and dead skin buildup and make it easier to thoroughly clean the scalp during shampooing. Remember, over combing or over brushing generally will cause damage to the hair, which is □uite contrary to the old 100-stroke brushing rule.

3. Avoid Excessive shampoing

Although clean hair is desirable and even necessary for the maintenance of healthy hair, excessive shampooing can strip vital minerals like calcium, phosphorus, nitrogen and iron from the hair. This is particularly true when using commercial shampoos. Most commercial shampoos contain formaldehyde as a preservative. To disguise the presence of formaldehyde it is listed in the ingredients as Quanternium-15. This substance can be carcinogenic (cancer-causing) and poisonous to the entire system. Unfortunately for those who suffer with dandruff, anti-dandruff shampoos are some of the most dangerous shampoos on the market. Selenium sulfide is the main ingredient in most dandruff shampoos, a substance that has shown to cause degeneration of the liver.

Other toxic chemicals such as polyvinyl pyrrlidone plastic (PVP), which is a proven carcinogenic, and creosol which has been proven to be highly toxic are commonly found in dandruff shampoos. This is why it is very important to correct this condition as □uickly as possible through natural means.

Natural shampoos normally found in health food stores are a much better choice. Even with natural shampoos, be careful of the ingredient Sodium Lauryl Sulfate can strip away too much oil from the hair, causing shampoo residue to be left behind. Ingredients that have proven useful in shampoos are cocamides, Panthenol Pro-B, of course the previously discussed vitamins, aloe vera, sage, nettle, burdock, chamomile, chaparral, horsetail and rosemary. Also look for shampoos that contain keratin, the protein substance that hair is made of, or amino acids. This will help seal breakages in the cuticle.

Choose a shampoo with a proper pH balance; a level of 5.5 is ideal. The pH scale runs from 0 to 6.9 for acids and 7.1 to 14 for alkaline, with 7 being neutral. Although generally conditioners are good for hair provided that they do not contain the previously mentioned harmful chemicals, shampoos with conditioners included should be avoided. Shampooing and conditioning serve two different functions and the effectiveness of both are diminished by combining the process.

When shampooing, pour the shampoo into the hands and rub the shampoo in with your hands rather than pouring it on your head. By pouring shampoo directly into the hair you may promote buildup in one particular spot. Massage gently with your fingertips to loosen flakes and buildup and to stimulate circulation, but avoid using the fingernails as this may scratch the scalp and cause scarring over time. Shampoo with warm water to open the pores and rinse with cool water to promote shrinking the pores back to their normal size. After washing hair, dry it by blotting the hair with a towel. Avoid rubbing, especially with terrycloth towels, as this will pull hair when it is in a weakened state due to the wetness.

4. Avoid excessive perms and relaxers

Be sure to follow directions on all perms and relaxers, as misuse can cause serious damage to the hair shaft. Excessive coloring, styling or heat treatments, and chemical treatments can damage hair and cause breakage even when directions are followed. Always keep in mind that these perms and relaxers have harsh chemicals in them that chemically alter hair, and long-term use of these chemicals can cause harm to hair shafts and follicles causing some hair loss. If you can avoid the use of these chemicals, by all means do. The result could be the increased life of your hair.

If you decide to use perms or relaxers to process hair, be sure to use semi- permanent hair color or henna. This will avoid harsh reactions between the relaxer or perm and the ammonia and peroxide amounts in permanent dyes. It is always best to allow the hair to rest untreated as much as possible, and avoid mixing chemical processes.

5. Avoid overuse of hairstyles

Another styling caution is against the overuse of hairstyles that pull the hair too tight, such as ponytails and braids, which will cause hair loss especially along the sides of the scalp. This syndrome is called traction alopecia. Keep in mind when styling hair that hair is living and growing, and is susceptible to the stress of constant pulling continuous abuse causes scarring, which will lead to permanent hair loss in the areas affected. Along with leaving the hair chemically untreated for a time, leaving it in a loose style without over-manipulation for as long as possible will ensure optimum results.

Chapter 5 - Black Hair Basics

The typical hair and hair follicles of those of African descent are tightly curled, thus producing hair that spirals. Black hair also typically has a larger diameter than Caucasian hair and retains less water, thus its relative "kinkiness." The many styling methods utilized on Black hair cause concern with hair loss. Black hair is very strong, fortunately so because Black hair styles cause a great deal of stress on the hair and scalp.

For example, using a hair pick to pick the hair up to a bushy style is a very damaging process due to the constant pulling causing stress on the hair shaft as well as the follicle. In fact, combing Black hair in general can create high stress on Black hair and cause breakage, which perpetuates dryness. Conrowing and braiding are methods of hairstyling that pull the hair tight, and this can cause a great deal of stress on the hair and scalp resulting in hair loss. Braiding that results in the hair being pulled very tight can cause traumatic alopecia, a hair loss that is caused by trauma to the hair and scalp. Traumatic alopecia is usually reversible with proper hair care.

Hot combs and relaxers used to straighten hair can cause a great deal of heat and chemical damage to hair and scalp, which can also cause traumatic alopecia, and over time can cause permanent hair loss. This becomes especially true when the heat or chemically processed hair is pulled tight by rollers or a hot curling iron.

Hot oil conditioners are excellent for Black hair, as hot oil treatments contain proteins and polymers vital to repairing the hair cuticles. Hot oil treatments involve heating the oil and putting it into the hair and scalp, then covering the hair with a plastic cap to allow the oil to soak in. Follow the recommendations on the treatment you are using for the amount of time you should leave the treatment on the hair. This process can heal breakages and shinier stronger hair will be the result.

Consider that hair relaxers commonly used on Black hair contain lye or similar chemicals that break down the hair shaft. Left on beyond the recommended time, these chemicals would eat right through the hair and cause it to fall out in clumps. This is why these same products are used in products like Drano® to clean clogged drains which often are clogged by hair.

No-lye relaxers are very popular today, mainly because it leads people to believe that the product is not caustic. This is far from the truth. The combination of calcium hydroxide and guanidine carbonate are combined to form guanidine hydroxide, which could just as easily clean a sink. Repeated use of such products can cause some degree of hair loss, and if scarring occurs while using these chemicals, the hair loss can be permanent in that area of the scalp. One must ask themselves is it wise to place such caustic chemicals in the hair on a regular basis for the sake of desired appearance? The question must be answered by each individual, however the facts should be known.

There is little that can be done to alleviate this syndrome without changing the typical hairstyles of African Americans. There is a catch-22 concerning relaxing Black hair, since combing natural Black hair causes so much stress and breakage of hair, while chemicals cause so much harm to the hair and scalp as well.

There are a few hair-relaxing products on the market that use chemicals and are somewhat less harsh than sodium hydroxide (lye) or its popular equivalent in "no-lye" relaxers: calcium hydroxide (quicklime) mixed with guanidine carbonate. One such product is called Natural-Laxer® and Sahara Clay® by Baka ProductsTM that has been on the market since 1990. This product is all natural and because it does not contain many of the harsh chemicals of commercial relaxers and actually contains only a finely ground plant called Daphne Gnidium and clay from Africa it is figured to be relatively safe. Of course this product does not straighten hair in most instances the same way as commercial relaxers, however it does tend to make Black hair more manageable. There is yet another product on the market that is reported to be 92-96% natural which is called Naturalaxer Kit In A Jar™ that does not require the applicant to comb through the hair during the application, which results in a lot less damage.

Of course the bottom line is once again, if you can leave your hair in its natural state then you will experience less stress and damage to the hair and thus prevent at least one cause of hair loss. There is a growing segment of the Black population that is becoming comfortable with wearing their hair in natural styles. One such style is dreadlocks. There are many rumors and myths concerning dreadlocks, as there is little proper information available concerning this style, and as with anything that is misunderstood many myths arise around it. Dreadlocks can and must be washed; otherwise they will smell badly like any other dirty hair. The best process to use to wash dreadlocks is to use a residue-free shampoo. Most commercially made shampoos leave residue and can cause hair not to lock, lending fuel to the rumor that hair had to be dirty to form dreadlocks. Clean hair actually locks much better than dirty hair, as dirt is a residue in itself that will inhibit hair from locking. For best results one should use a fragrance free, conditioner free shampoo. Dreadlocks do not react well to oily and greasy substances, yet there are many good substances that are on the market today that will assist you in forming dreadlocks. Dreadlocks are formed through a process, not simply by not combing or brushing the hair. Generally, one should start with hair about two inches in length, and the hair should be separated into even squares of hair and twisted gently together using a bonding or gel substance. Many use natural beeswax containing no petroleum, while others use loc and twist gels specifically formulated for locks. Once the hair is separated and twisted into small locks, it is important that they are left alone and allowed to bond naturally. The length of time it will take to lock will depend on the coarseness of your hair, but one can normally expect to wait several months before locks begin to form. While the hair is locking, it will need to be washed. Here is where washing should be extended for a while if possible, so that the hair can be allowed to lock for two weeks to about a month without manipulation. When you do wash your hair, use a stocking cap or "do-rag", and low-pressure water to make sure that the newly forming locks do not come loose. It will be necessary to rinse for a much longer time than you normally do, because of the lower pressure of the water and the lack of direct manipulation of your hair with your hands. The water is good for your hair and locking process, so this is not a problem. It is also imperative as indicated before that you use a shampoo that does not contain a conditioner and leaves as little residue as possible. A little research on your part will be necessary here; your health food store should contain a variety of natural shampoos. Have a skilled professional or a friend re-twist the hair gently, reapplying the twist gel or beeswax that you used previously. Repeat this process every two weeks to a month, the longer you are able to wait the better, and within a few months your hair will begin to lock.

Again, if you have a fine grade of hair rather than a kinky grade of hair, a beautician skilled at forming locks ("locktitian") or a friend who is very familiar with the hairstyle should be consulted. Even though dreadlocks are mainly a hairstyle for Blacks, there are other races that have people that enjoy the hairstyle. In general, it tends to be a style of hair that in the long run will give the hair and scalp needed rest from the rigors of chemical and heat treatments and rigorous combing and brushing, and therefore can contribute to longer life for your hair.

Chapter 6 - Hair and Scalp Diseases

There are a variety of hair and scalp diseases; some are very common, while other more severe hair and scalp diseases are fortunately rare.

1. Alopecia Areata

Alopecia Areata is an autoimmune skin disease that causes the body's immune system to attack the hair follicles, causing baldness in patches. It affects 1.7 percent of the population, including 4.7 million people in the United States. In cases where the disease progresses to the point where all scalp hair is lost, it is called Alopecia Totalis, and where hair loss advances to the entire body it is called Alopecia Universialis. There is no known cause for alopecia areata and therefore no known cure. The disease usually hits before age 20, and does not seem to favor one particular gender or culture. Hair loss with alopecia areata comes in stages, with hair returning and falling out in phases. For information on this disease, contact the National Alopecia Areata Foundation (NAAF) at PO Box 150760, San Rafael, CA 94915-0760, (415) 472-3780.

2. Seborrheic Dermatitis

Seborrheic Dermatitis, an advanced form of seborrhea, is a non-contagious skin disease that causes excessive oiliness of the skin, most commonly in the scalp, caused by overproduction of sebum, the substance produced by the body to lubricate the skin where hair follicles are present. Seborrhea is the form of the disease where oiliness only occurs without redness and scaling. The disease commonly occurs in infants, middle-aged people, and the elderly, and is commonly known in infants as cradle cap. The disease has no cure, yet in infants it usually disappears in time. With adults the condition may persist with varying degrees of severity. Flaking, scaling and redness often are symptoms of this disease. It is easily treated with topical solutions found in creams containing corticosteroids and shampoos containing pine tar, selenium sulfide or salicylic acid. Seborrhea and seborrheic dermatitis are both easily treated and controlled, and should be because left untreated they can contribute to hair loss. In fact, a group of Japanese scientists have linked the overproduction of sebum to hair loss. This is because the sebaceous glands in areas of the scalp where hair is thinning or bald are enlarged, and are thought to cause the clogging of pores and several other problems that promote hair loss.

3. Psoriasis

Psoriasis is termed an immune-mediated disorder that affects different areas and functions of the body. It is non-contagious, and one of the areas of the body it can affect is the scalp. It usually appears as patches of raised red skin accompanied by burning and itching. Several contributing factors are thought to contribute to the outbreak of psoriasis, including emotional stress, certain infections, toxemia, the thinning of the intestinal walls and adverse reactions to certain drugs. At least half of people who have psoriasis have scalp psoriasis. Like seborrhea, scalp psoriasis left untreated can cause hair loss. Fortunately, it can also be treated with a variety of topical creams and shampoos containing tar and salicylic acid. For more information on psoriasis, contact the National Psoriasis Foundation at 6600 SW 92nd Ave., Suite 300, Portland, OR 97223-7195, (503) 244-7404 or (800) 723-9166.

It is vital not to scratch the scalp and pick at the scabs that psoriasis causes, as this could damage the hair follicles in the dermis and cause permanent hair loss. As long as the follicles are not damaged, hair loss caused by this malady is usually temporary and hair will grow back once the condition clears. Some of the best ways to stop the itching are using very common household substances such as mouthwashes like Lavoris®

and Listerine®. Carbolated Vaseline® works well along the hairline to relieve symptoms. Hair dyes of all kinds and chemical treatments such as permanents and relaxers should be avoided at all costs with psoriasis. These chemicals are extremely harmful in general, but with psoriasis can lead to irreversible damage to the hair follicle over a relatively short period of time.

Like any of these other maladies, one must keep in mind that psoriasis cannot be cured through drugs, and if any cure exists it is in the form of the body healing itself by the correction of malfunctions in the body. One condition present with everyone suffering with psoriasis is toxemia. When the body becomes toxic, various genetic dispositions mature and psoriasis is but one illness that arises due to toxemia. Toxemia is caused by poor circulation and the thinning of the intestinal walls. The patient's blood becomes acidic, and thus this acidity comes through the largest organ in the body: the skin.

a. Several cases of psoriasis have been healed through natural processes such as internal cleansing, giving up alcohol, increasing the intake of water-especially distilled water, an increase in exposure to the sun in certain cases, an active reduction in stress by removing stressful conditions and practicing meditation, and the elimination of nightshades such as tomatoes, tobacco, eggplant, white potatoes, peppers (not black pepper) and paprika.

b. One food that is a common plague to those suffering with psoriasis is pizza. Obviously containing tomatoes, pizza also contains every ingredient a psoriasis sufferer should avoid, such as white flour, peppers and hot spices. Additionally, pizza is highly acidic and should be avoided by all means.

c. In addition to the dietary suggestions given earlier, it is suggested that those suffering with psoriasis should eat fish, poultry and lamb regularly, maintain a high alkaline diet and consume low fat milk or buttermilk. Fish, especially fresh or canned salmon, sardines and solid white albacore tuna contains Omega-3 fatty acids that are vital for skin and scalp health. Although most fish are recommended, avoid dark-fleshed fishes such as mackerel or bluefish, sushi or shellfish. Poultry such as chicken, turkey, Cornish Hens and other non-fatty fowl are excellent foods for those with psoriasis when not fried. To avoid excess fat, remove the skin before eating and avoid fowl that has high fat content like goose and duck. Lamb is the only recommended red meat for those suffering with psoriasis, being that it is easy to digest and still a great source of protein. Of course it should be prepared any way except by frying.

d. Dairy products should be consumed sparingly, and only low-fat or non-fat dairy products Those suffering with psoriasis can obtain their calcium from sources mentioned earlier in the section on Diet, Nutrition and Hair Loss, such as soybean products, celery, lettuce and greens.

e. White bread should be avoided. And a limited amount of whole grain bread and whole grain products can be substituted, but should be consumed with caution because all grains except millet are acid forming.

f. Additionally, one should eliminate alcohol consumption entirely, except for perhaps a small glass of red wine with dinner to promote rich blood and digestion.

g. For cleansing suggestions, see the earlier section on Natural Hair Loss Remedies. Lecithin is beneficial for psoriasis, and can be taken in its granular form in the dosage of one tablespoon three times a day, five days a week, either plain or added to water, juice, sprinkled on salad or cereal. After the condition clears, reduce the dosage to one tablespoon taken once per day, five days a week. Lecithin can be obtained at any health food store, and although it can be obtained in li□uid or tablet form in addition to granular form, it is best used in granular form due to the high phosphatide content when consumed as such. These doses should not be exceeded, as the over consumption of lecithin can cause a blockage in the absorption of calcium

4. Eczema

Eczema is another non-contagious skin disease that mimics psoriasis very closely. Eczema produces scales, reddened inflamed skin that periodically ooze, and the familiar itch that is of supreme annoyance to those that suffer with it. These are however two different diseases that usually re□uire different treatments. However, there are certain treatments that work for psoriasis that work for eczema also. Eczema causes extreme buildup and sores on the scalp, and can cause severe scarring. The buildup caused by eczema can cause temporary hair loss, however the scarring that can occur especially if one scratches the painfully itchy lesions can cause permanent damage to the hair follicles.

Eczema is an illness caused by toxemia as well. And although one can use the various medicated shampoos and creams on the market to control its symptoms, permanent relief is only going to come from removing the cause of the toxemia. Therefore once again cleansing and drinking plenty of purified water are keys to fighting eczema. Many of the dietary recommendations are the same for one who suffers from eczema, except there is usually an increased sensitivity to fish-therefore it should be eaten in a limited amount. Also, there is usually a high intolerance of cow's milk, since eczema is highly associated with allergies. Therefore, one should use soymilk or goat's milk instead.

5. Hair Loss due to Chemotherapy

Hair loss due to chemotherapy treatments is a common side effect of the treatment. Chemotherapy kills rapidly reproducing cancer cells, however the side effect of this treatment is that chemotherapy also destroys the rapidly reproducing cells that promote the growth of hair and nails. Hair is lost rapidly and in large ☐uantities in most instances. During this process, no prescription, herbal or over the counter treatments of any kind have been found to assist in maintaining the hair. Fortunately, hair normally returns within six months to a year after treatments cease. Patients have found that hair re-grown after chemotherapy is finer in texture and lighter in color at first. These are usually temporary conditions that improve with time. Those recovering from chemotherapy should avoid chemical processes such as perms, relaxers, bleaching and coloring in the hair until it grows at least three inches and not until at least one year after the last treatment. Chemotherapy can cause skin sensitivity and these chemicals can be extremely irritating to the scalp.

6. Women's Issues

The term Male Pattern Baldness (MPB) tends to lay credence to the thought that hair loss is primarily a male problem. While males do lose hair more readily and tend to lose hair in sections, women suffer baldness and hair thinning also, except the thinning is more uniform throughout the head. With this is mind, women are better candidates for surgical hair replacement and weaving treatments, because large portions of the scalp are highly unlikely to be bald on a woman suffering with androgenetic alopecia. Because a great deal more emphasis is put on the beauty of a woman's hair, this is becoming a great concern for today's woman.

While the general information covered thus far is good for all persons in general, there are a few things specific to women concerning hair loss.

Many women suffer hair loss and an increase of facial hair after the onset of menopause. This is because of the drop in estrogen production, changing the ratio of estrogen to testosterone in a woman's body. Prior to menopause, a woman's body is constantly producing estrogen, which binds excess testosterone to proteins called globulins. Therefore, there is little excess testosterone in a woman's body. After the onset of menopause this estrogen is no longer present, thereby exposing it to a similar although milder type of syndrome that males go through concerning the overproduction of DHT.

An interesting note is that once again, the syndrome of menopause and its unique effects are not as common in the Eastern world, but are specific to Western civilization. The key differences are the consumption of less red meat and fatty foods in Eastern lands than in the West and less daily stressors in most Eastern lands as compared to Western civilization. Anorexia is an eating disorder that is becoming more prevalent among women in the past few decades and is psychologically driven in Western society due to the emphasis put on slender women being the ideal in Western civilization. Needless to say, if you or a loved one is suffering with this disorder, a qualified physician should treat any cases of anorexia. However, some of the side effects of anorexia can be hair loss due to the malnutrition the syndrome caused. In this case, it is vital to carefully follow the advice given in the sections Nutrition, Diet, and Hair Loss, and Natural Hair Remedies.

It is of course recommended in all cases that you reduce your intake of red meats, fatty foods, and reduce stress, however due to your profession and engrained habits there may be a limit to how much you can change this part of your lifestyle. There is another factor in Eastern civilizations that may cause a stark difference in their women not suffering through typical menopausal symptoms here in the West.

The consumption of soybeans and soybean products is much higher in the East. This is significant because soy contains estrogen-like substances and work in the body similarly to estrogen. Therefore there is not an extreme drop in estrogen levels in women who consume soybean products, thus reducing the symptoms of menopause typically suffered in the West. Some women who suffer hair loss tend to have gastrointestinal problems that do not allow them to absorb proteins and zinc that are necessary to maintain a healthy head of hair. If you think that you have problems with your gastrointestinal system and are experiencing unusual hair loss, of course see your doctor. You may be able to take some natural non-dairy acidophilus after meals for a couple of months in order to increase your digestion of these nutrients.

There are a number of myths associated with hair loss in women particularly. Many were told that brushing the hair 100 strokes each night will promote healthy hair growth. As mentioned earlier, extreme brushing of the hair can cause stress on the hair which can cause breakage and hair loss. Also, just as hats have been rumored to cause hair loss, wearing wigs has also been rumored to cause hair loss. This is very untrue, especially if the scalp is given sufficient time to breathe at night and hair is washed regularly to avoid buildup.

Although stress can cause temporary hair loss, permanent hair loss is usually unconnected to stress. Last but not least, the belief that there are cosmetic products that are out on the market that grow hair is simply unfounded. There is only one product on the market that has been proven to grow hair on women safely, and that is women's Rogaine® discussed later in the section Over The Counter Treatments.

During pregnancy hair growth increases dramatically in most women. This increases the usual percentage of hair normally growing on the head. Therefore, after childbirth there may be an increase in hair loss due to more hair follicles than usual entering the rest phase. The temporary excessive loss of hair usually occurs between one and three months after childbirth and is quite normal; it should balance out a few months after childbirth at most. Similar syndromes occur after ceasing birth control pills or switching types of birth control pills.

Chapter 7 – Hair Replacement and Restoration Techniques

There has been a great deal of progress in the field of hair replacement and restoration in the past few years. Surgical techniques have improved greatly from the days when hair replacement first began. All hair replacement techniques involve the use of your own hair; therefore, hair replacement candidates must have some healthy hair, usually at the back and sides of the head. The process is a relatively safe procedure when performed by a qualified surgeon, however as with any surgery there are risks. Candidates must be checked for uncontrolled high blood pressure, blood-clotting problems, or skin that scars excessively, as these conditions may make healing difficult. Small pieces of hair growing scalp grafts are removed from areas of the scalp with healthy hair and are placed where hair is thinning. There are three major types of grafts:

a) punch grafts

Punch grafting takes about 10-15 hairs and places them in the scalp. This was the first type of technique to be developed, and when first developed caused a patchy look in many candidates. The technique has been improved since the first days of being developed, and the new mini-graft technique has also been added as an option.

b) mini-grafts

Mini-grafts contain only 2-4 hairs per graft, and therefore look much more natural.

c) micro-grafts.

Micro-grafts are still smaller grafts that contain one to two hairs each. To maintain healthy circulation of the scalp, grafts are placed 1/8th of an inch apart.

Local anesthesia is usually sufficient for these procedures, and several procedures are usually required to achieve the desired result. Post-surgery, a period of approximately 10 days of no sexual or strenuous activity is recommended, as strenuous activity may cause bleeding from the graft areas. Of course surgery is a serious option, and often an expensive one as well. For those not wishing to undergo surgery for either reason, the option of non-surgical hair additions is often explored. Many professionals have developed techniques to add hair to existing hair on your scalp that look very natural.

Techniques for Bonding hair to existing Scalp

Weaves, fusions, bonding, cabling and micro linking are some of the techniques used to bond hair to the existing hair or scalp non-surgically.

1. Toupees & Wigs

Many jokes were made in the past about wigs and toupees, and they have gained an unfavorable light amongst many people because they were so obvious on the wearer. Today's toupees and wigs are often made of real hair and are very well styled, causing them to look more natural on the wearer. These hairpieces are held in place by affixing adhesive to the scalp and stay in place through vigorous exercise. Of course you will need to seek a professionally made toupee in order to make it worth your while, and you should purchase at least two so that you can maintain them properly, servicing one while wearing the other. A professionally styled and fitted toupee is expected to cost upward of $600 to $1000 in today's market. Of course no one wants to go through the embarrassment of wearing the obvious "rug" on top of your head, so if you are not willing to spend the money it takes to purchase a professional toupee then it is probably best to not wear any hairpiece at all. Structured hairpieces as they are called are a semi-surgical approach that permanently attaches hair to the scalp by stitching the hair to the bald scalp. This procedure is not recommended, as it is a process that involves introducing a foreign material to the scalp. Most ethical surgeons do not perform this procedure any longer as they are generally deemed to be ethically inappropriate. If this procedure is recommended to you, get a second opinion from a trusted physician.

2. Hair Weaving

A much safer procedure is hair weaving, yet this can only be used if hair is thinning and large balding areas are not present. The process is also called hair intensification or hair integration. Strands of synthetic or real hair are braided or weaved into your own existing hair giving an appearance of a full head of hair. This procedure does have its drawbacks, because it can make the scalp difficult to access, interfering with proper hair and scalp maintenance necessary for the health of your remaining natural hair, and this method can also stress existing hair since the artificial hair introduced through weaving is attached to it. This method is usually expensive, costing several thousand dollars per application, and being that because of the aforementioned drawbacks it can only be left in for a few weeks at a time it is usually impractical for the average person. It is highly recommended that one seek professional assistance with these procedures from licensed beauticians or barbers, and have a patch test done to the skin if using adhesives to test for skin sensitivities. Extra care must be taken to maintain cleanliness of the hair and scalp when wearing added hair in order to maintain the health of existing hair and the scalp in general. Of course, if you are undergoing chemotherapy or are in the early stages of diagnosed alopecia areata then these procedures should be avoided as the hair they are connected to is likely to fall out as well. Either waiting for a period of time or obtaining a full prosthesis is recommended in these cases.

3. Spraying Micro Fibers

Yet still there is another type of treatment which is a spray of micro fibers made up of the same substance that hair is made of: keratin. If your hair is simply thinning, while you are investigating a more permanent solution to your hair loss problems or in the process of employing a particular process that takes some time, you can use these substances to cosmetically produce the appearance of thicker and fuller hair. The substance is marketed under several different names, one such being Topik®. Being a temporary solution it is relatively inexpensive, and can provide some immediate aesthetic results to bolster confidence and optimism as you work on more permanent solutions.

Chapter 8 - Medical Treatments

Over The Counter Treatments

The most popular over-the-counter hair restoration drug today is Rogaine®, a brand of topical monoxidil solution by Pfizer Corporation, approved for over the counter sale in 1997 by the Food and Drug Administration (FDA). Monoxidil was originally used as a blood pressure medication, and then doctors found that it produced the side effect of increased scalp hair growth.

Today monoxidil remains the only FDA approved pharmaceutical topical solution proven to grow hair. In the preliminary studies held in 1985, 55% of men tested were able to re-grow hair with extra strength Rogaine® (5% topical monoxidil treatment), although the best results came from those who had been balding for less than 10 years and were bald in a section of four inches across or less. Another test study compared the results of regular strength Rogaine® (2% topical monoxidil solution) with the extra strength version, and found that subjects grew 45% more hair with the extra strength Rogaine® than with the regular strength Rogaine®, and users of both solutions outgrew the users of the placebo. Only 6% of those tested experienced any type of irritation.

Rogaine® works by blocking the production of DHT. Of course there are generic brands of topical monoxidil solution also on the market. Rogaine® was originally made only for men's use, and then a women's version of the drug was produced. Similar results were achieved with the women's version. As with both men's and women's versions, users must take note that continuous use of the drug is necessary to maintain the newly grown hair, as it is a usual reaction for newly growing hair to stop growing and fall out when one ceases to use the drug. As with any drug, follow all directions and cease to use if irritation or discomfort persists. Of course many people choose not to use drugs to treat conditions, because they want to avoid the use of chemicals and their possible side effects. In this case, there are several treatments in existence that have been found to block the production of DHT and thus work similarly to topical monoxidil products.

As mentioned earlier, Saw Palmetto has been used effectively to block DHT in the treatment of prostatic disease, and is now being explored for its effectiveness in stimulating hair growth. Traditionally it has been used by herbalists to stimulate hair growth effectively. Nettles, usually taken in the form of Nettle Root Extract has shown itself to be effective in preventing hair loss as well. More information on these was covered in the section called Natural Hair Remedies.

Prescription Drug Treatments

While topical solutions such as Rogaine® brand monoxidil have been used to treat hair loss, Propecia® brand Finasteride by Merck & Company, Inc. is the only FDA approved pill approved for the prevention of hair loss and possible hair re-growth. Like Rogaine®, Propecia® was discovered when its generic e□uivalent being used for another purpose was found to have beneficial side effects.

Finasteride is the generic name for the drug, which was already in existence for □uite some time and had been produced under the name Proscar® by Merck & Company and used for treatment of enlarged prostates, a syndrome medically called benign prostatic hyperplasia (BPH). BPH is caused by an overproduction of DHT, which causes the prostate to grow. Many BHP patients were also suffering with MPB, and when patients began taking Proscar®, they noticed the re-growth of hair also. This sparked new testing and the birth of Propecia® as a hair restoration drug. The approval of Propecia® by the FDA was easy to achieve, since it was merely marketing already approved Finasteride as a hair restoration drug, with a much smaller dosage than that re□uired for BPH.

Propecia® is being prescribed by doctors to some patients as an oral treatment to internally block the production of DHT. Propecia is an androgen hormone inhibitor only approved for men, and has been clinically proven to grow hair on a significant percentage of men who suffer with Male Pattern Baldness (MPB) or more properly androgenetic alopecia. Unfortunately, the drug has not been approved for use by women at this time. This is especially true for women who are pregnant or can become pregnant, because the process of inhibiting testosterone from being converted to DHT can affect secondary sex characteristics of unborn fetuses.

Propecia® works by reversing the shrinkage of hair follicles that are in the telogen phase, or last phase of the normal hair cycle. Propecia® works best in combination with topical treatments of Monoxidil such as Rogaine®. Participants in studies have seen hair grow in as little as six months, whereas those who have seen no results in a year's time are reported not likely to see any results from the drug. One round of testing of over 2,000 men with androgenetic alopecia over a four-year period showed half with reported new hair growth. Side effects of Propecia® in a few persons studied include diminished sex drive, difficulty in achieving an erection, and a decreased sperm production. Side effects were found in less than three percent of participants in clinical studies. Fortunately when the drug's use was discontinued, the side effects went away and normal functions resumed. Of course there are some who say that the growth of new hair is worth the cost of a drop in libido. Only you can decide whether this side effect is worth the personal cost to you.

Finasteride is metabolized primarily by the liver, and therefore anyone suffering with liver disease may not be able to take the drug, and should consult a physician. Additionally, as with Monoxidil, it can mask PSA levels, thus caution should be used if used by patients with elevated PSA levels, as it may be difficult to read levels properly when diagnosing potential prostate cancer. Of course proper consultation with your physician will help determine if taking Finasteride treatments such as Propecia® is right for you.

An interesting phenomena concerning Propecia® is the dramatic rise in price it caused for Finasteride when it entered the market as a hair restoration drug. Propecia® is simply a 1mg version of Finasteride, a drug that was already being marketed as Proscar® for BPH by the same company that markets Propecia®, Merck & Company, Inc. Therefore there should not be an increase of any kind in the cost of production of Finasteride, since it was simply being marketed under a new name at a much smaller dosage. Merck & Company therefore was prepared to introduce Propecia at the price of $1.25 per pill or $37.50 for a

30-day supply in 1998. However, after reconsiderations it was decided that Propecia would be introduced at $50 for a one-month supply. This is compared to a 30-day supply of Proscar® which is 5mg Finasteride being marketed at $55-60.00 for a 30-day supply. The price was adjusted to be in the range of Rogaine® Extra Strength. While Proscar® prices have risen at a much slower pace, and is now less expensive than the same Finasteride drug that is 1/5th the dosage. Doctors of course are discouraged by pharmaceutical companies to prescribe Proscar for cosmetic treatment of androgenetic alopecia. Of course there are always going to be those who find ways to circumvent this. Therefore, many have been driven to find ways to purchase Proscar® and divide the pill into fourths or fifths instead of paying the exorbitant prices for the very same Finasteride.

Conclusion

Hair is a living protein, and as with any living part of our bodies we must be sure to maintain proper health to optimize our chances of maintaining a healthy head of hair. Proper nutrition is vital to maintaining healthy hair, since the hair is a living and growing part of the body's system. Viewing it in this manner can help us to treat our bodies different and raise expectations through proper care. A healthy balanced diet, occasionally with the help of vitamin and mineral supplements and exercise are all key components to a healthy regimen of maintaining healthy hair.

Male Pattern Baldness (MPB) or androgenetic alopecia is the condition that over 95% of persons that suffer hair loss have, and it is caused by a rise in DHT, a direct component of testosterone. The scientific developments of the past two decades have brought hope and promise to many who suffer with this type of hair loss. Treatments like Rogaine®, Rogaine® for Women, Propecia, and improved surgical treatments have brought relief to many who would have previously had to settle for gradual hair loss, wigs, or hairpieces. The discovery of the role of DHT in preventing hair loss has even opened the doors to possible herbal solutions to hair loss prevention, such as saw palmetto, nettles, rosemary and horsetail. Even more promising is the fact that the hair loss commonly known as androgenetic alopecia is found to occur mainly in Western civilization or those who have adopted the ways of Western civilization, meaning that there may be dietary practices that contribute to hair loss and therefore giving hope to the possibility that diet could control not only temporary hair loss, but androgenetic alopecia as well.

Doctors and scientists are studying DHT production in the body to understand it more thoroughly. There is an obvious link to hair loss and prostatic health and this only increases the pace of hair loss discoveries. Most treatments for prostatic diseases such as benign prostatic hyperplasia (BPH) also have the pleasant side affect of growing hair on the heads of those taking it. With the pace of research and discoveries today, there is a great deal of optimism in the field of hair loss prevention. Hair is an important part of our dress and appearance, therefore a large part of our self-esteem. It is likely that there are answers for your situation presently or coming in the near future.

Remember, the restoration of hair growth is not an overnight process. The process takes time regardless of the method chosen. Be patient and follow as much of the advice given by professionals as possible. Keep in mind that the body is a system, and it is the abuse of this system by food intake and environmental causes that lead to most common hair loss. Through returning the body back to its natural state, hair growth can be restored. Good health to you!

Thank you again for purchasing this book!

I hope this book was able to help you realize that food addiction is not a hopeless case and that there are effective treatments that can help you overcome it.

The next step is to try to follow the advice and tips in this book to help you stop the hair loss. Remember that there are thousands of people in the world who are in the same situation as you are. You are not alone.

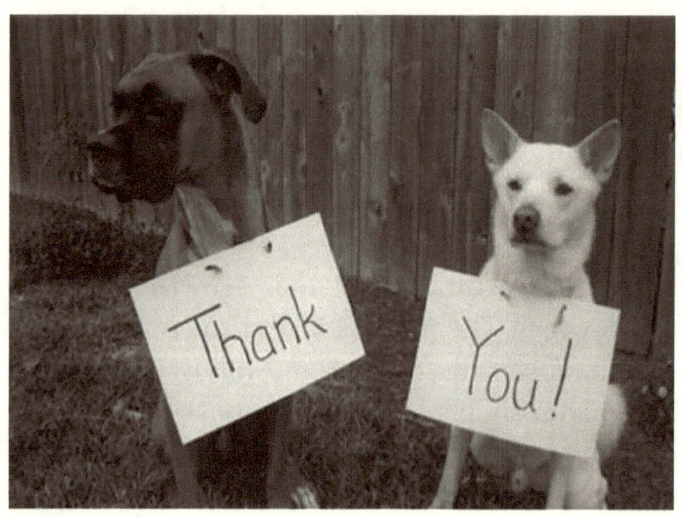

Finally, if you enjoyed this book, please take the time to share your thoughts and post a review on Amazon. It'd be greatly appreciated!

Thank you and good luck!

Check Out My Other Books

Below you'll find some of my other popular books that are popular on Amazon and Kindle as well. Simply click on the links below to check them out. Alternatively, you can visit my author page on Amazon to see other work done by me. If the links do not work, for whatever reason, you can simply search for these titles on the Amazon website to find them.

1) The Ultimate Guide To Overcome Anger - How To Manage Your Anger Before It Controls You

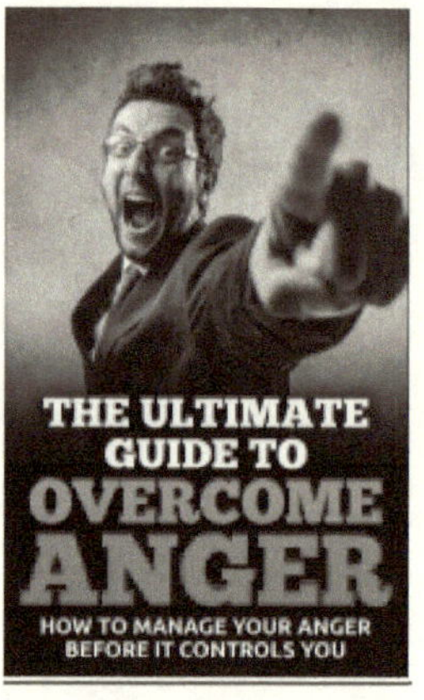

go to: http://amzn.to/1Pzm3Yy

2) The Ultimate Guide To Become An Alpha Male - How To Attract Women, Win In Life And Be Confident

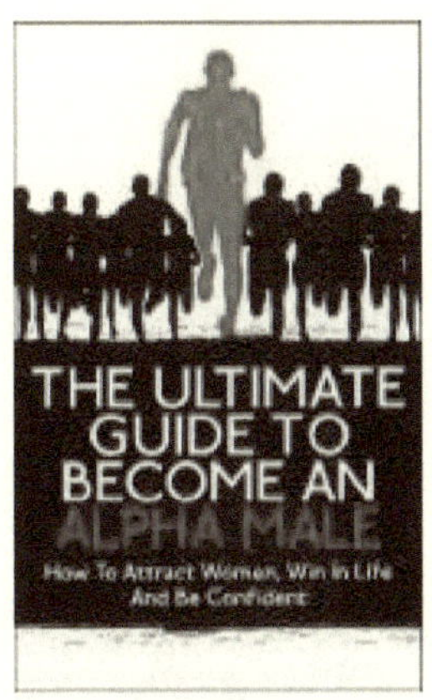

go to: http://amzn.to/20G8bBo

3) The Ultimate Guide To Overcome Porn Addiction For Life - The Most Effective, Permanent Solution To Finally Stop Porn Addiction

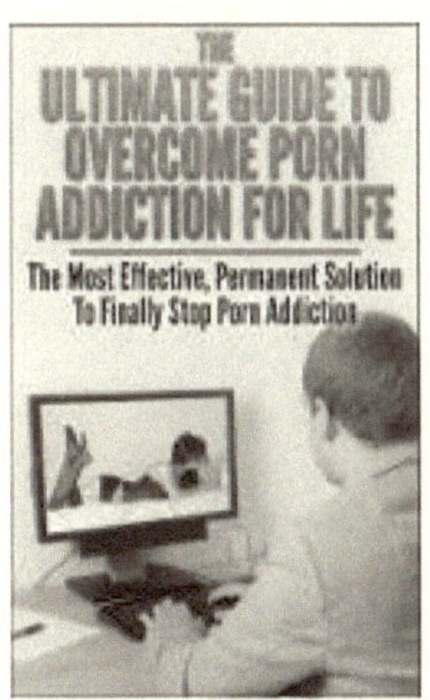

go to: http://amzn.to/1NZ2tmN

4) The Drug Addiction Cure - The Most Effective, Permanent Solution to Finally Overcome Drug Addiction for Life

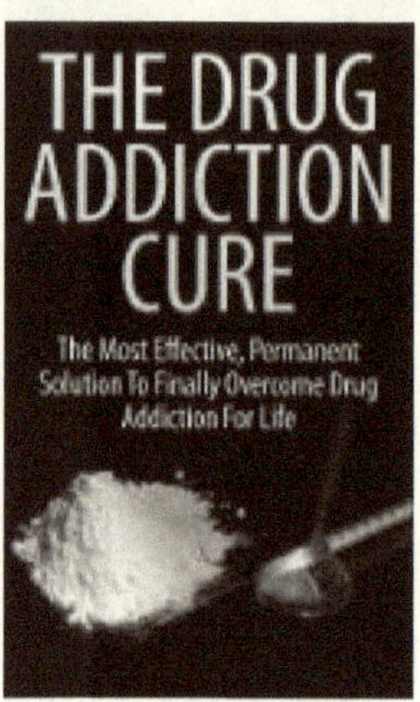

go to: http://amzn.to/1kkb9uc

5) How to Stop Snoring for Life - The Most Effective Cures and Remedies for Snoring

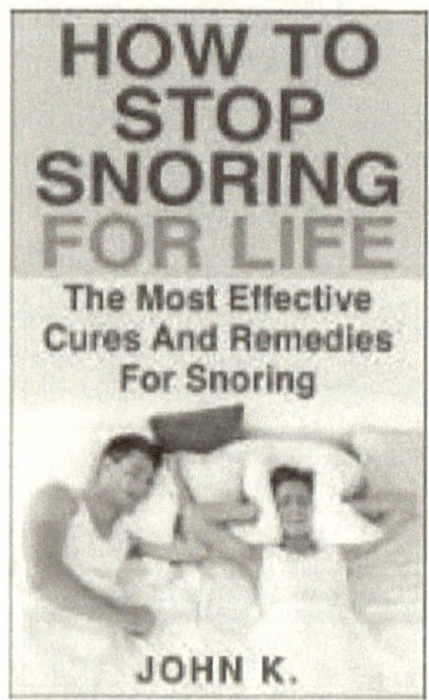

go to: http://amzn.to/1NE9uLn

6) India - The Land of Mystery, Mysticism, Mythology, Miracles, Multiculturalism, and Mightiness

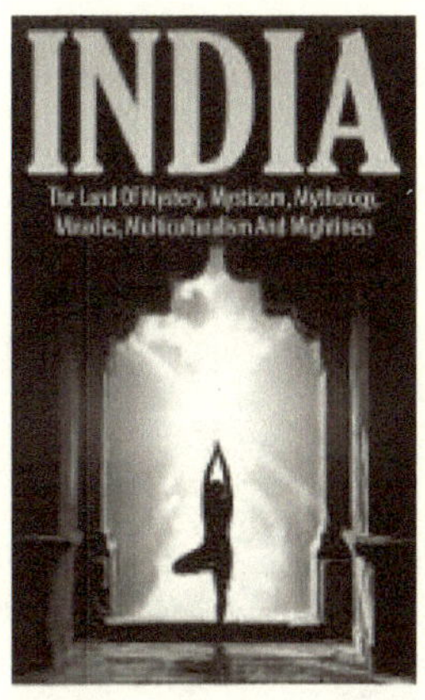

go to: http://amzn.to/1kkbBc5

7) The Ultimate Guide To Become An Early Riser For Life - How To Awake Early And Be Productive Forever

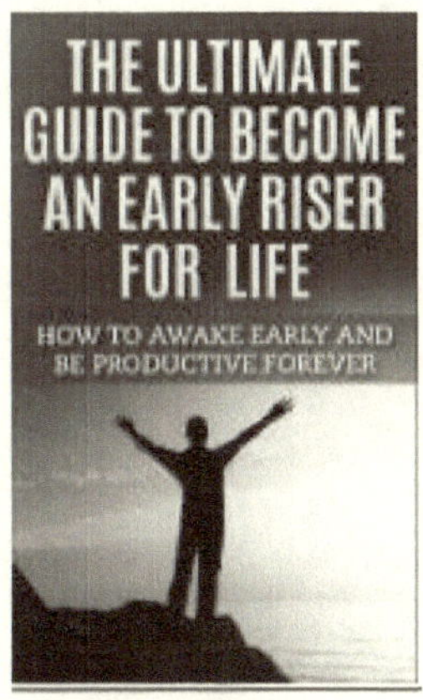

go to: http://amzn.to/1MRDEMr

8) The Ultimate Guide To Overcome Rejection - How To Get Back To Life After A Rejection

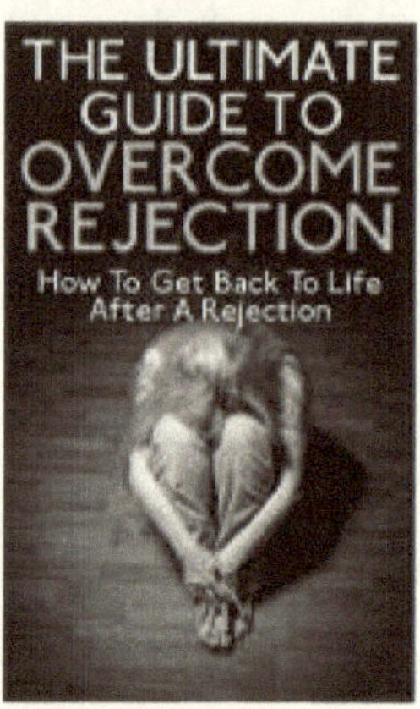

go to: http://amzn.to/1M1xMMZ

9) The Ultimate Guide To Overcome Marijuana Addiction -

The Most Effective, Permanent Solution To Finally Cure Marijuana Addiction For Life

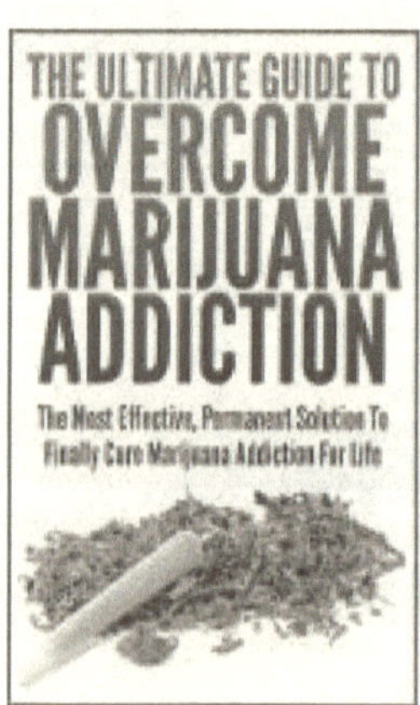

go to: http://amzn.to/1M1xQMN

10) The Ultimate Guide To Overcoming Shopping Addiction

- The Most Effective, Permanent Solution To Finally Control Compulsive Shopping and Buying Disorder

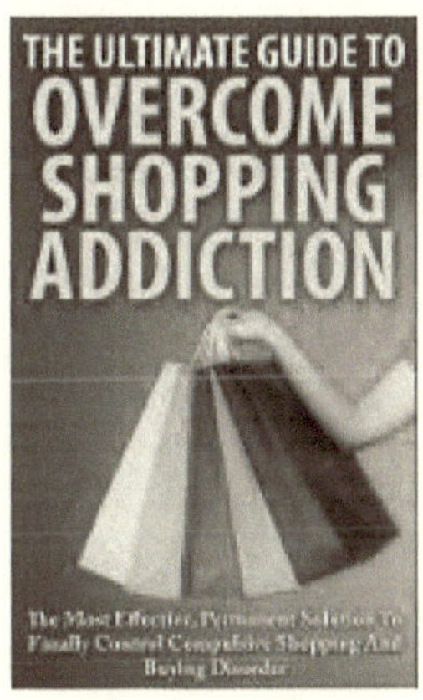

go to: http://amzn.to/1L6oiJr